Immune System Boosters

Build a Bulletproof Immune System with these All-Natural Boosters

Nora Roth

Table of Contents

Introduction

The Immune System: A Quick Look At What Makes It Tick

Taking Charge: Can You Really Boost Your Immune System?

Getting To Know Your Immune System

10 Ways You Might Be Weakening Your Immune System Right Now

Creating a Bullet-Proof Immune System

Top 10 Immune boosting Foods

   Should You Buy Organic?

Top 10 Immune Boosting Vitamins & Supplements

Exercise For Building Your Immune System

   Personalizing and Exercise Program

Finding Relief from Stress

Secrets of a Good Nights Sleep

Conclusion

Copyright © 2015
All Rights Reserved

You may not reproduce, store in a retrieval system, or pass on in any form or by any means, electronic, mechanical, photocopying, recording, scanning, or otherwise, except as allowed under Sections 107 or 108 of the 1976 United States Copyright Act, without the prior written permission of the Publisher and Author, any material in this guide.

TERMS AND CONDITIONS

The information contained in this guide is for information purposes only, and may not apply to your situation. The author, publisher, distributor and provider provide no warranty about the content or accuracy of content enclosed. Information contained herein is subjective. Keep this in mind when reviewing this guide.

The information in this guide is not provided as medical advice. You should always consult with your doctor if you have a health condition that requires treatment. The authors, publishers and owners of this guide are not medical doctors, psychologists or psychotherapists of any kind, and are not qualified to provide medical, psychological or therapeutic advice. You agree to hold all parties associated with creation and sales of this guide free from liability associated with any physical, mental, emotional, psychological or other harm arising from use of this guide or the website.

Neither the Publisher nor Author shall be liable for any loss of profit or any other commercial damages resulting from use of this guide. All links are for information purposes only. We do not warrant for content, accuracy or any other implied or explicit purpose.

INTRODUCTION

Life is unpredictable. We cannot control the curve balls it will throw our way. That's simply impossible. But, we can control, to some extent at least, what happens inside our bodies. We have the power to take charge of more than we may think we do. By maintaining a healthy diet, exercising and doing other beneficial things for ourselves, our bodies are much more likely to be in top performance. After all, our bodies are a direct reflection of our inner health.

Neglecting bodies, like eating junk food and simply not taking care of ourselves, we are asking for trouble. In not washing our hands, we risk all sorts of germ-borne illnesses. We often just give in to illnesses that float around in the winter months, hopelessly giving in to them. But the truth is, that is simply not true. We can do much to stay well.

You have probably heard miraculous tales of chronically ill patients who have overcome their disease. They refused to give in and took matters into their own hands. In doing so, they took charge of their destiny.

Why leave your health in the hands of fate when you have the power to change it?

THE IMMUNE SYSTEM: A QUICK LOOK AT WHAT MAKES IT TICK

Diseases are always lurking. Illnesses come at all seasons of the year. It doesn't make any difference what time of year it is, your body is constantly vulnerable to such things as viruses, influenza and the common cold. At any given time, you can end up with food poisoning or a number of other maladies too. Everywhere you go, disease is lurking. But don't worry, that doesn't mean you have no power to control disease. You can pump up your immune system by taking some simple, yet powerful steps.

Before getting to the steps of boosting your immune, it is vital to learn how you actually become ill and how disease works. As you get a feel for how it all works, it will begin to make sense to you. That is when you can take hold of your body's defenses and change the entire course.

What conditions make you more likely to get sick in the first place? The winter is a time of year that is notorious for illnesses of all kinds. One reason for that is the amount of time people usually spend indoors. It's cold out and so people stay in, making germs more likely to be passed around. It has also been noted that because people are often less active during the winter time, they are more likely to sit around doing nothing which leaves the body apt to get sick due to lack of exercise.

Even for those who ventilate their homes from germs and keep in tip top shape throughout the cold months are not exempt from getting sick. But there is a good chance they won't get as sick.

Even the warm summer months carry their fair share of illnesses. On the positive side, the immune system within our bodies stand guard and are always ready to defend against and wage war on foreign invasions. That is, of course, unless you suffer from an autoimmune disorder or for some reason your immune system is compromised. That is why even those who opt not to take medication for a cold will get over it in a week or so.

Even if you do have a condition that compromises your immune system, a disease does not have to get the best of you. You still have the option to fight back. And...you should. Of course you will want to talk to your physician about the exact nature of your illness and what is best in your particular case.

When it comes to illnesses, there are a lot of different root causes. Viruses can be causes by bacteria. Bacteria is generally successfully treated with antibiotics. Unlike viral illnesses, bacterial ones are usually eliminated with antibiotic. Knowing the root of your sickness will help you in finding the cure.

The Truth About Antibiotics: Should You Take Them?

Antibiotics have become the "go to" for whatever ails you. But, is this wise? While many people are under the misconception that antibiotics are a cure all for any and every illness, this is simply not true.

There are a good number of antibiotics that are able to wipe out many diseases, they cannot sure them all. Antibiotics do not work to rid the body of viruses, only of bacteria. It is imperative to distinguish which is at the source of your illness in order to find the proper solution.

When you have a viral infection, you will not get help from taking an antibiotic. In fact, quite the contrary. If you do take them, your body is likely to build up those antibodies causing the next round of antibiotics you are given for a bacterial infection to not work like they should. In applying the wrong solution, you can make matters drastically worse.

Bacteria are pro at adapting. They are like chameleons, camouflaging themselves to mimic their surroundings. They are sneaky too. They change as they grow and mature. Thus, they can easily disguise themselves and then they gain power and control. That is the reason that some antibiotics are no longer effective in areas where they once were and also is why there are a small number of antibiotics that can take on some diseases that are more dangerous.

The overuse of antibiotics is a real problem. It's become an epidemic. Many physicians tend to over-prescribe them because they feel undo pressure to do so. Many patients are guilty of asking for them, or demanding them because they simply want to feel better, quickly. They long for instant relief.

The patient often feels better after taking the antibiotic due to the fact that their bodies have had just enough time to start fighting the illness off. It appears that the antibiotic is helping when in fact, it's is just time that is the healer.

It's a serious and often overlooked subject. Antibiotics are dangerous and not something to take lightly. If there is any way that you can avoid taking them…do so.

That should shed a better light on just how imperative it is to understand the prevention of illness and how we may be doing things to harm our bodies' ability to fight off disease by thinking we are doing the right thing.

Taking Charge: Can You Really Boost Your Immune System?

Know that it is more possible than you may think to take measures to help your body be less likely to get a cold or at least to help ensure that you will get over it faster and not be affected as severely by it. This book will help give you tools to combat not only the common cold but also bacterial diseases, flu, illnesses that are food born and many others as well. Do remember to check with your doctor or healthcare professional when you are sick.

Rest assured that we are in no way trying to take the place of your doctor or healthcare professional. In fact, quite the contrary. They are the authority when it comes to your health. The mission of the guide is to give you relevant information and helpful hints that will assist you in your quest for good health and the prevention of getting sick. Please be sure that if you are taking any kind of medication at all or are in treatment for any illness or chronic disease, you speak to your doctor before using any of the tips in this book.

Much has gone into this book. It is accumulation of years of research that entails the mind, body and spirit and the connection between them. It is by discovering the causes at the root of the illness that we are more able to find the cures. Rather than merely treating the symptom, our goal is to get to the heart of the matter. To do that, it is necessary to reinforce the mind, body and spirit and the harmony between them. You will be amazed at the connection.

Ideally, each of the bodies' systems works together and in doing so, helps keep your from disease. There are things that you can do in order to encourage the systems to be in one accord. Then, there are things that will be beyond your control. You can infuse your home, office and car with aroma therapy essential oils but you most likely cannot place them in each and every place you go to. That is why it is important to do what you can where you can. Everyone is unique therefore what works well for one may not help another at all so find out what methods are helpful to you and stick with the winners.

Before we go any further, please note that before attempting to treat or cure an illness, you should always seek medical advice.

Take it to the top. Your doctor is the one who is qualified to treat an illness and diagnose it as well. He can distinguish between a bacterial and a viral infection. There are many realms your health care professional should be a part of so keep that in mind, please.

Now for the tools that you can use to combat illness and to boost your immune system. When it comes to health, there is no given. There is no guarantee that comes along with these suggestions and what works for one may not work for another. However, the techniques are found to be beneficial by many who have learned how to stay well or, at the worst, shorten the duration and strength of an illness.

Take note. There are sections of this book that you may want to write down. You may even want to create a list of things to do in order to optimize the information. Whatever you need to do in order to make the most of this guide, do it. It will be "well" worth your while!

Getting To Know Your Immune System

When you get a better knowledge of how your immune system operates, you will understand the entire process better. To do so, you can use several methods including visualization and meditation to enable your body to defend against disease better, no matter what the source of it is.

The immune system is the center of our health and well-being. You can't function fully without being in good health. Generally, our immune systems obey our bodies' commands. They fight diseases and ward off bacteria too. How does it all work though? Keep reading to find out the answer to that very important question. You may be surprised to learn how simple it all is.

Imagine, if you will, a body that has been perfectly and thoroughly taken care of. It would be a powerhouse for fighting against disease of any form. It would be way stronger than any antibiotic or antioxidant on earth. What if we followed our gut-driven instinct to gather and consume foods that are really optimal for our health and cared for ourselves as we do for others, no longer putting our own selves last? The results would be astounding. The reality is that most of us don't care for our bodies near like we should and leave ourselves wide open for disaster.

Fighting Infection and Disease: It's Only Natural

Just how do our bodies fight off infection and disease? It's really amazing how it works. It all begins when bacteria or virus germs find their way into your body. There are a myriad of ways they do this and simply washing your hands does not immunize you from them although it does help.

The examples below will show you in just a few steps what takes place when disease first comes into your body.

1) Most germs spread by contact. When you touch something, are showered by a sneeze or come into contact with something unclean, germs, like bacteria and viruses can enter your body. Did you know that one cough may spread phlegm up to 500 feet away? That hones in the fact that everyone should cover their mouth when coughing. But the fact is, many don't.

2) The red alert is actually white. When your body encounters problems, the immune system shoots out a message that it is time to bump up the production of white blood cells. White blood cells fight off infections that cause disease no matter if they are bacterial or viral.

3) Springing into action, infection fighting antibodies are produced as well, helping to fight off not only infections but allergies and various other disorders too. There are more than one type of antibodies. IgE help to combat allergies while IgA goes after infections.

4) Warfare begins with a vengeance. Your body sends ample antibodies and white blood cells to fight any attack, no matter how severe. This doesn't mean you won't get sick, it means your body will do everything it can to keep you healthy. If you get sick, the chances are high you will recover much faster if your immune system is working well.

5) While those with average immunities may have a "bug" for 7 to 10 days, those whose immunities are compromised may take much longer to recover.

Realistically speaking, it's a given that the normal person does not have an immune system that is in tip-top shape. Chances are that you don't either of you would not be reading this guide. You will learn, though, the tools to use in order to get it into shape though. You will have a better chance of not catching something or at least shortening the duration and lessening the severity. There are many factors that come into play when working with the immune system, what makes it tick and what makes it malfunction and you are about to learn about those.

10 Ways You Might Be Weakening Your Immune System Right Now

There are a number of ways in which your immune system may be threatened. Below are some things that may be behind your bodies' failure to combat infection or disease.

Don't forget that even if you just have one of these habits, there is still a negative pull and your immunity can be compromised. Your chances of a poor immune system greatens when you are guilty of two of these and so on.

1. **Saturated fat** - Fat is a real threat because it clogs your arteries and also can help to cause type II diabetes and of course, adds pounds that can cause issues as well. Fast foods are high in saturated fats and processed food is horrible for your body as well.

2. **Lack of exercise / exercise intensity -** Exercise is a fantastic tool to use to bump up your immune system but only if done correctly. Too much, too quick will drive your body into a state where it is actually backfiring and your immunity will go down. Exercise but do it wisely

3. **Stress levels are too high -** Stress gives way to many health issues such as heart attacks, depression, high blood pressure and a myriad of other conditions. You will be better able to fight disease when you rid your life of excessive stress.

4. **Lack of sleep -** Those who are sleep deprived tend to eat more and also are prone to get sick more often.

5. **Too much sleep -** When it comes to sleep, balance is key. Sleeping in excess of 10 hours per day, health issues are sure to surface. If you are doing so, be sure to see your physician who can check for underlying causes. Six to eight hours a day is the

average amount most people can operate on but 7 to 8 is optimal

6. **Unbalanced eating habits** - Moderation is the answer to the problem when it comes to eating. If you starve yourself, your body will go into a survival starvation mode and you will slow down your metabolism which means that you will gain weight instead. It will put an undo load on your immune system as well. The best thing you can do is eat small portions of good, healthy foods.

7. **Bad Habits-** Smoking cigarettes, drinking too much alcohol and other indulgent activities will leave your body much more vulnerable to disease. Bringing foreign substance into your body risks free radical damage. Free radicals are cells that are on a mission to steal, kill and destroy. They can set off a chain reaction and the result is often illness and disease. Be careful what you put into your body and what you expose it to.

8. **Lack of Common Sense-** Sometimes we do things we know are not smart. We go out in the freezing cold with our hair wet or stay in the sun until we are fried. Even going around people we know are sick puts us in the position to get sick. We put our bodies in situations that tax it and then, we pay the price. By using common sense, we can avoid compromising our immune system beyond what it can handle.

9. **Thinking Yourself Sick-** It is a fact that what you think is what you are. If you are just sure you are going to catch the illness that has made its round throughout the office, you can bet that you will. Have you ever NOT come down with what everyone else has because you knew you could not miss a day of work or because you had something important coming up? You really can talk yourself into getting sick…or, not getting sick.

10. **Hygiene Matters-** Since germs generally enter the body through contact, you can prevent many from entering your system by

frequent washing of your hands and also by sanitizing things that you come into contact with that are likely to be touched like doorknobs, public phones and light switches. When shopping, take advantage of the sanitizing wipes that are by the grocery cart and wipe off anything you will be touching.

While it may seem a little high-tech, fine tuning your body like you would a complex machine is the way to go. Just as you put oil in your car, you need to put food fuel in your body, and it needs to be of good quality.

The more you care for and respect your body, the better your overall immunity system will work. Doing otherwise will surely show. You can get by with cutting corners on many things in life but your health is not one of those things. Treat your body with the utmost care and it will do you well. Treat it poorly and it will do the same. Good health is well worth investing in.

Next is learning the steps that will lead you to optimal health and the maximum immunity you are searching for. Following these steps will help you attain a happy, healthy and prosperous future. Are you ready for the challenge? If so, keep reading to find out how to do it.

Creating a Bullet-Proof Immune System

When it comes to protecting your body against intruders like colds, the flu and other illnesses that are often experienced by the very old and the very young, your immune system is your best defense. If you aren't eating right and taking care of yourself in general, you will most likely be compromised and catch whatever comes your way.

If you are lacking in the area of optimal health, you can learn how to change that and live a healthier lifestyle.

There are many ways you can boost you your immune system including:
- Basic hygiene
- Foods

- Herbs
- Vitamins and Supplements
- Exercise
- And more…

So let's just right into it, shall we?

KEEPING YOUR HANDS CLEAN

It sounds too simple but the very first step to a strong immune system is to wash your hands, wash them often and wash them well. If you don't have access to a good old fashioned sink to wash your hands often you should carry a bottle of natural hand sanitizer to take its place

The top reason people get sick is via hand-to-hand contact. Shaking hands, touching door knobs and even holding your child's hand can give germs a direct path into your body. You come into contact with germs and then forget to wash your hands before you eat or touch your lips and…you are exposed.

There are things you do without even thinking that can be very bad habits when it comes to acquiring germs. Be sure that you are washing your hands often and that those in your household are doing so as well, especially when someone has a cold or is sick. You should wash your hands during these critical times, for sure. If you want to decrease your chances of getting sick, these are some times where it is critical for you to wash your hands.

1. **When going to the gym** – Going to the gym is a must for a healthy immune system but there are lots of people sweating it out on those machines.
2. **At Church** – If you go to church like I do, everyone wants to shake hands. And while that's great for fellowship it's not so great for spreading germs.
3. **Anytime you are around lots of people.** If you are out and about where there are many people, this is even more important.
4. **When going out to eat**. Anytime that you venture out to eat, be it a fast food chain or a sit down restaurant, be certain to wash your hands good before you indulge. If you don't have access to running water and soap, you can resort to a moist towelette or hand sanitizer.

5. **When caring for someone who is sick.** It's easy to forget about our own health when caring for someone who is ill. Remember though that you can spread the germs when you fail to wash up after touching someone who is sick or something that they touched.
6. **Taking the kids to the park.** Don't forget to bring moist towlettes if nothing else when you go to the park, especially if you are going for a picnic. Pass them around so everyone can use them. Individual bottles of hand sanitizers are good to bring along and use too. A tiny bit in your palm will go a long way and may save you from a world of germs.

7. **When handling pets.** Our pets are often like family to us. They become children to many. But don't forget that they can carry diseases so be sure to wash up when you have come in contact with your pet or anything they have come into contact with.

8. **Before preparing food.** When handling food, you for sure need to wash your hands. Whether you are cooking the food or

serving it, be certain you scrub up before doing so. If you don't, you could spread germs to all who partake of the food. Meat and vegetables should be treated even more cautiously. Even cutting them on a cutting board without cleaning it in between can create a breeding ground for germs.

9. **When handling money.** Yes, money is said to be the root of all evil and it is the root of many germs as well. When you have handled money, be it change or bills, be certain to wash up as money is passed through many hands and carries a multitude of germs.

10. **When pumping gasoline.** Who would think the simple act of pumping gasoline into your vehicle could be the source of illness? Many hands touch the handle of gas pumps and truth be known, most are rarely, if ever, sanitized.

Top 10 Immune boosting Foods

For boosting the immune, there are a number of foods that will help do so. While they don't cure a cold or ailment, they certainly can help your body fight harder against getting sick and even help lessen and shorten symptoms if you do get sick. Scientific studies have proven that chicken soup lowers white blood cell activity and therefore really does help.

Nature has much to offer when it comes to fighting off illness. What are good foods to eat when sick or fighting getting sick? Which should be avoided? The foods below are likely to boost your overall health and wellness and make it more possible for your body to defend when infections or viruses attack.

1. **Water** – Before getting to far into foods there is no double you need more water! Studies show that the body's need for hydration can be mimicked by the feeling of hunger. It sounds absurd but it is a proven fact that overeating is a symptom of simply being overly thirsty. When water is purified from chemicals, it is about the best substance you can put into your body. It can help you not get sick and can help you get better fast if

you do. People in dry climates tend to get dehydrated. Water is a must for keeping the digestive track on track and for keeping disease at bay so...drink up!

In addition, water benefits your skin and works to keep it healthy and also assists your entire body in washing out toxins so it will help keep you in good health. If you are not a huge water fan, try adding lemon, lime or another flavoring to it. It is a fact that those who are dehydrated actually do not get very thirsty as a rule so the more you drink water, the more you will want it.

2. **Tea** – many teas have a wealth of antioxidants packed into them and green tea is no exception. Not only does it help boost your immune, it is soothing too. Black tea is another that is very beneficial but green tea takes first place in this contest. Green tea is also said to work alongside your body's metabolism, promoting it to help you shed pounds. So next time you are

feeling under the weather, you might try a steaming cup of green tea with a squirt of lemon in it.

3. **Flax or Fish**– essential fatty acids are very small substances that assist the body to reduce inflammation which is plays a large role in illnesses. Of course you can take Omega-3 fatty acid supplements, but you can also add them into your food intake. Mackerel, salmon and tuna fish are some foods loaded with essential fatty acids.

4. **Yogurt** – yogurt helps to control and balance the flora that dwells within your digestive organs. When your flora level is out of control, diseases can abound like yeast infections, urinary tract infections and many others as well. Make sure to look for a real yogurt with live cultures. Not something artificially sweetened and full of chemicals.

5. **Mushrooms** – Believe it or not, medical practitioners from the Far East eat

Shitake mushrooms to boost immunities. Why is that? Vitamin B among other essential vitamins and minerals can be found in mushrooms in general. Although the exact amount of essential nutrients vary in the different varieties of mushrooms, most have some and can be beneficial to fight sickness. Shitake mushrooms are my favorite for immune system.

6. **Fresh fruits** – we've all heard the saying, "An apple a day keeps the doctor away." Fruits do actually help the body resist disease. Bananas, y blueberries, raspberries and strawberries are at the top of the list when it comes to bolstering immunes. The reason is that they are rich in antioxidants which play a key role in fighting illness at the root of the cause. They wage war on free radicals which are cells that are on a mission to destroy. In addition, fruits have various other beneficial nutrients such as bananas have potassium, which aid in balancing your body with electrolytes.

7. **Help From the Ocean-** People from Eastern civilizations have eaten seaweed in their diet for hundreds of years. Seaweed is thought to pump up the activity of T cells which combat disease and illnesses. It is also thought that seaweed helps the body in the production of antibodies, the white blood cells that lend themselves to fighting off infection and diseases. Oysters have been recognized as being effective at combating illness too.

8. **Herbs** – not only do herbs add flavor to your favorite dishes, they also help ward off diseases. Cumin, cayenne, cilantro and oregano are among the most powerful. Cayenne is said to heat the body and spur many healing benefits by doing so like increasing metabolism which even assists in weight loss. Don't leave out herbs when it comes to bolstering your immune system.

9. **Onion and Garlic**– both onion and fresh garlic are great for immunities. You can take them in supplement form or eat them right out of the garden. They are powerful sources to help keep you well. Garlic is an antibacterial, antifungal and also gives you energy. It works wonders when combined with onion in soups to release nasal congestion and also to get immunities flowing.

10. **Whole Grains** – Barley, Oats and other whole grains are chalked full of fiber and are great sources of antioxidants and antimicrobials. Research shows that both oats and barley may rev up the body's natural immune system and help to combat things such as the flu. .

While of course this list does not go into all the foods that can help you stay well, it does cover some of the top ones. One great rule of thumb worth mentioning is to avoid processed foods when possible. They not only contain preservatives but are generally high in fat content as well. Even those that are fortified are not optimal. Fresh is best when it comes to food.

When foods are eaten in their original state or "whole", they are much better for you. Fruits, vegetables and grains can all be found in whole. Nature supplies disease fighting ingredients in our food supply. It is when we alter the food that it loses the ability to help us out in that area.

Meat that does not contain any antibiotics is best and milk is optimal with no hormones. It's the same rule as with fruits, vegetables and grains. The less it is altered, the better.

Milk is generally pasteurized which is understandable but it does lend itself to the hormones and antibiotics that were given to the cow. Therefore, if you or your child drinks milk, you also drink the hormones and antibiotics. There is speculation that adolescents these days are going into puberty earlier.

Should You Buy Organic?

There is a shift going on these days. More people are learning just how bad chemical ridden foods can be. They are also learning the value of eating nutritious, unaltered, whole foods.

Walk into the produce department of most any grocery store and you will notice some things new things are happening. Many are offering more organic and whole foods in place of processed, traditional food.

Now, you are presented with a choice. Buy organic or non-organic. But what exactly is the difference besides the price tag?

The majority of organic foods are grown on farms that are organic. Heavy chemicals and pesticides are not allowed if the farm is certified organic. There are no hormones given or no enhancement of size, shape, etc. No GMO's are used either. .

So while your tomato may not be as large as the non-organic one it sits beside in the produce section, there is good reason. It is a product of nature, not of man. It may even be a little odd in shape but that is from the natural process of growing it. The good thing is that with organic, you and your family are not ingesting or chemicals.

There is an influx of people who are becoming more and more aware of organic foods. While some are fans due to the taste, others are sold because there are no chemicals in them. They do tend to cost a bit more. If you are limited in funds, you might try a few organic varieties here and there and also, there are often times samples that are available. Co-ops and farmers' markets are a more affordable way to shop organically and you might even consider growing your own. If you do grow your own, check into organic seeds because it is defeating the purpose if you use seeds that are not free of chemicals including GMO's.

More information about farmers' markets and co-ops can be found online. You can sometimes visit the locations and find out more.

Here are some helpful links:

http://coopdirectory.org
http://localharvest.org
http://organicconsumers.org/purelink.html

There are services that will prepare and deliver organic foods straight to your front door. Some also deliver boxed goods that supply you with a number of organic products.

A service that I really like is:
http://DoortoDoorOrganics (use coupon code "fitness" for a discount on your first order)

Online you will find pre-cooked meals available.. Here is a site that offers that service:
www.theorganicdish.com

The organic food service is quite similar to other food services like Weight Watchers. But, with this particular one, your ingredients are all organic. The phone book and local organizations It's almost like any other prepared food service, like weight watchers, however with this program you get organic ingredients and meals delivered right to your door. You might try searching your local phone book for information on a service like this too as they are becoming more and more popular as the public is shifting from chemical-laden foods to organic.

Top 10 Immune Boosting Vitamins & Supplements

You just can't beat eating healthy. It is crucial to your well-being and general health. But, it is also wise to take vitamins and supplements. Sometimes we just need more nutrients than we are getting. That is when taking a supplement can help fill in the gaps.

Do be sure to speak to your health care provider before doing so though. If you take prescription medications on a regular basis, you need to be sure that supplements do not counteract each other or cause side-effects. That is why it is imperative to speak to your doctor before taking any. You can get information and advice for a qualified healthcare provider or of course, you can do your own homework and make your own call on the matter.

As far as supplements go, here is a list of some of the most popular ones that are recommended for bolstering the immune system:

1. **Probiotics** – probiotics are also called "acidophilus" or other substances which relate to the role probiotics in helping the body balance natural (good) flora and get rid of bacteria that is residing. Good bacteria is essential for the body to eliminate wastes and digest properly. When you take an antibiotic prescription, it not only gets rid of the bad but of the good too. There is research that suggests that when probiotics are taken, the risk of digestive diseases subsides and they also

increase the immunity factor within the body.

2. **Oregano oil** – Oil of oregano is known as *"nature's most powerful antibiotic"* Personally I do 3-5 drops of oil of oregano every morning. I drink it with 20 oz. of water and lemon juice from half a lemon.

3. **Omega-3 fatty acid** – you can purchase omega-3 supplements like fish oil or flax seed oil that will actually benefit your entire health and well-being. Since essential fatty acids assist in reducing inflammation, doctors often prescribe it to arthritis patients and other diseases that come with swelling and inflammation.

4. **Vitamin C** – inexpensive and effective, vitamin C is one best ways to spruce up your immune system. As mentioned, there is a lot of controversy regarding how much is needed but sift through the

information and also consult your physician and you should find an amount that is right for you. Personally I suggest a whole food vitamin C *(stemming from something like camu camu or acerola cherries).*

5. **Medicinal mushrooms** – Mushrooms are powerful immune system boosters but surprisingly very little known. Shitake is a great mushroom or there are many mushroom blends you can use to boost your immune system. Check your local Whole Foods or Vitamin Shoppe to see what they have available.

6. **Echinacea** – this is a universal herb known to help with many ailments. When ingested at regular intervals while you are experiencing a col, it very well may help reduce the duration as well as the severity of it. It is available in capsules and in tincture formulas. While it is not generally recommended to take it all the time throughout the year due to

its possibly loss of potency and effectiveness in your system, it is often suggested that it can greatly help during the peak of cold and flu seasons.

7. **Goldenseal** – this herb is very potent that it should be used with caution. The antibacterial and antiseptic contents in it are so powerful, they can upset your stomach and even cause pregnant women to experience contractions. But taken within reason and when needed, it can greatly help you stay or get well. Consulting a physician or herbalist is recommended.

8. **Zinc** – often overlooked, zinc deficiencies are behind many symptoms of tiredness and fatigue. It also helps to remedy the symptoms of a cold and is found in many cold formulas because of that fact. Zinc is one thing that is commonly lacking in our diet so it is a good one to take as a supplement. There are also zinc lozenges that can be purchased and those are very

soothing to sore throats and good for bolstering the immune.

9. **Colloidal Silver** – this mineral has been used throughout history to combat disease including such serious ones as the Bubonic Plague. In the solution, silver particles are suspended in liquid. It is the silver ions that are effective in destroying bacteria and are sought after for their medicinal qualities. Colloidal Silver can be toxic though and too much of it can turn your skin blue so he sure to speak to your doctor before taking this mineral.

10. **Vitamin D-** Vitamin D is super effective to boost your immunities. Eating foods rich in D can certainly help you battle disease and you can also take it in a supplement and catch some sun rays as well.

There are lots of products that claim to benefit your health and keep you from getting sick. Some do. Some don't. There are some that contain a blend of vitamins and minerals and many get the formula just right. Others add fillers in and don't use quality ingredients to begin with. An herbalist can direct you to the right shelf if you are having trouble deciding between supplements and herbs and mixtures. The assistance of someone who knows what they are doing and knows about basic drug interactions and so forth is good to have to help you.

While you are looking into supplements, herbs and the likes, you may want to ask about prevention remedies like Shitake mushrooms and garlic. These are most useful when taken in the quest to avoid getting sick.

One great way to pump up your natural ability to fight disease is to use plenty of garlic in your diet. You can take a capsule and you can also you it as flavoring on your food. Garlic is akin to goldenseal in that it is a very potent and natural antibiotic. It, like goldenseal, may upset your stomach if you ingest too much so be careful. There are some modern versions of garlic supplements that are tasteless and odorless too which is a huge plus.

Knowing more about supplements that can boost your immunity system is a good start to great health. Now let's take a glance at the next two steps that can assist your body in wiping out disease.

EXERCISE FOR BUILDING YOUR IMMUNE SYSTEM

Exercise is a word dreaded by many but it's too important to leave out. Exercise is a good thing. It will help improve your health and assist in you not getting sick. The trick is to find something that interests you that also gives your body exercise. Play tennis or walk alongside the lake. Combining what you like to do with what you might not be so fond of (exercise) is a good way to make it more appealing.

To find out the optimal exercises for your particular situation, it is strongly advised that you consult with your physician. There are many factors to take into consideration when starting an exercise regime. Health condition, medications and age all play a factor. Even just a little exercise will help to bolster your immunity. So, do what you can.

Even if you have no need to lose weight, the fact is that you need to exercise too. The fact that you may be skinny doesn't mean you don't need to stay in shape so you can ward off sickness. In fact, many people who are thin actually carry around a good deal of fat within their bodies. The percent of body fat is what ultimately matters health-wise. Fat actually weighs less that muscle does so don't be deceived. You don't have to have a weight issue to have a reason to exercise.

For instance, if you weigh in at 120 pounds and are 14% lean, you will have a different appearance and a different health condition that someone with 30 % body fat who weighs exactly the same. .

Classification	Women (% fat)	Men (% fat)
Essential Fat	10-12%	2-4%
Athletes	14-20%	6-13%
Fitness	21-24%	14-17%
Acceptable	25-31%	18-25%

Obese   32%+   25%+

To find out if you fall within a healthy body fat range, check the following chart:

If you don't know your current body fat level you can usually get a "wellness evaluation" by a personal trainer or health coach in your local area for not much money.

If you just want to get an estimate of your body fat percentage without doing an evaluation I found a good image to help you do that at :

http://www.fitbodykitchen.com/body-fat-percentage/

Either way its good to know where your body fat currently is so you can make a plan to improve it. Having a healthy overall weight and body fat percentage is one the best things you can do for your immune system and your overall health.

Personalizing and Exercise Program

While there are a myriad of great exercises that will help you get your body in shape to fight off illness, there are some that are universal and most anyone can do them so let's focus on those.

Your current health, your age, your physical activity level and other factors will help to determine the type of exercises that best suit you. You can decide which are right for you. If you are extremely out of shape, you will want to start slow such as walking around the block whereas if you are used to running marathons, you will run instead.

The term "walking" is used loosely but it generally denotes a brisk walk when done as exercise. You want to get your heartrate up. That is the object of the game. Pumping or moving your arms while you walk will help achieve a higher heart rate. Again, do check with your doctor to be sure which things are right for you to do when it comes to exercising.

Your doctor can also give good advice on power walking and what additions you might add in or if you should not add any at all. Below are more exercises that can be done in moderation or full force. Again, get medical clearance before doing any of these.

1. **Yoga** – This low impact way to exercise is especially great for those with dexterity issues. It helps your body's ability to flex, is gentle and generally simple to do and cleanses the mind at the same time.

2. **Pilates** – This is an exercise that, like yoga, is very great for you and is a super way to enable the body to better resist disease. It is also excellet for balance and strength.

3. **Strength Training** – If you are out to lose fat and want to build and improve your muscle mass, this is exactly what you want to do. It might be easiest to begin on machines and then go on to free weights but the choice is yours. Do be certain to have someone coach you through this initially. You don't want to end up ripping a muscle.

4. **Swimming** – you work every group of muscles when you lightly swimming and it's

easy on your joints too. You don't even have to actually swim. You can do yoga in the pool or aerobics.

5. **Climbing Stairs** – if you have healthy and strong knees you may like climbing stairs for exercise. Stadium bleachers are usually not too hard to find and they are excellent to work out on

6. **Jogging and Walking**– Lots of people who start out walking end up as joggers once they build up to it. Be careful what you run on though. Soft ground like grass is easier on the joints that cement.

7. **Biking** – Many people enjoy biking outside. They love the challenges of the terrain and enjoying the fresh air. But if that is not practical for you due to weather or other reasons, you can always exercise on a stationary bike indoors.

8. **Tai Chi** – A practice having to do with meditation, this exercise is a lot like yoga but is actually easier on the body because it is done while standing with gentle postures

and little or no impact. It is said that Tai Chi restores the body's energy flows.

9. **Meditation** – It has been stated that if you are too busy to meditate, then you are…too busy. Meditation is well worth the time you put into it. Input equals output in this case. While there are those who do not feel like meditation qualifies as an exercise, others do. It gets the body, mind and soul into shape and that, they say, is exercise. Whether you feel it is justified in being considered one or not, you will most likely agree that it is beneficial for your health and therefore certainly worth doing. In addition, it has been proven to decrease stress which is a key contributing factor to disease. You may also find that you get twice as much done when your mind and body are at peace with one another.

10. **Visualization** – See the situation for what it is! This exercise is for the mind. Imagining yourself back to great health really is possible. You can picture your body fighting off sickness and create images of your

healthy body. Don't underestimate just how powerful the mind is. Seeing is...believing and in believing we conquer a multitude of evils.

Each and every day, your body, mind and spirit need exercise in order to survive and especially to thrive. Focusing on disease and illness will no doubt make you more susceptible to get them. Focusing on great health and combating disease will aid in your quest for stronger immunities. The concept of visualization is so powerful, in fact, it is used in many cancer centers.

Funny, but lighter and gentler motions that are done through Tai Chi, Yoga or Qigong which is a low-impact Eastern exercise which focuses on the movement of energy within the body are often more effective than rigorous ones. These passive exercises have been proven to boost immunity and also give the body a burst of energy. When you have more energy, you can more easily fight what is coming at you like a cold or a disease. Your chances of keeping an infection at bay are much better too. These exercises are easy and many enjoy doing them.

Visualization can be super effective and require little physical movement. You can picture disease and infection as being gone and focus on bacteria and virus being nipped in the bud. You can also see yourself as healthy and energetic and soon, you will being to feel a change for the better. When you see it, you believe it and that is the beginning of great things.

The subconscious is an incredible machine. It can "trick" your brain into projecting health simply by thinking you are healthy even if you are, in fact, not healthy at all. It sounds absurd and really, it is but it is reality. Many physicians use visualization to help their patients with a speedier recover and also to bring recovery at all to those who suffer with chronic illnesses.

It's mind over matter – literally!

Of course there are those who are against visualization. They think that it is a hoax. They feel it is like a placebo which is when one thinks there is change or improvement but there really isn't. When there are medical test done and it is a blind study, some are usually given a placebo, sugar pill. Sometimes those people feel as if they have improved or have had a positive change. There are many who do improve because they think they have…mind over matter.

While the placebo effect certainly does not occur with everyone, it may be an answer for you. If you believe it, it may come true. What do you have to lose?

Finding Relief from Stress

It's a fact that the less stress you have, the better you feel and the better you feel, the healthier you are as a rule. Stress is not a good thing at all. It is very destructive. It is one of the most common reasons you get sick and are unable to fight off disease. It impacts your life more than you may think.

Once reason that stress is so harmful is that stress makes it hard to get a good night's sleep. When that happens, then your body has great difficulty functioning properly. When your body doesn't function like it should, it is easy to get sick because your immune system is not at its best. If you want to bolster your immune system, getting proper rest is key.

Do you have any idea how much stress you are under?

Take this stress test:

In order to figure out where your stress triggers lay, or exactly how much stress you have inside you, here are some questions you might ask yourself. See how many of the following apply to you.

1. Do you feel lethargic or tired? Are you worn out during a day that follows a good night sleep? Do you ever wake up tired?

2. Do you worry Non-stop about such things as work, school, family or any other matters?

3. Are you constantly arriving to events late because you are trying to make up for work or obligations that you did not get accomplished due to putting them off? Do you tend to put more onto your plate than you can possibly chew? Do your overachieving tendencies get you into trouble when it comes to timeframes and deadlines?

4. Do you find yourself having too many alcoholic drinks too often in order to relax?

5. Do you experience bouts of excessive crying without reason, or feeling depressed much of the time? Are you often sad or overwhelmed with emotions?

6. Do you have a sense that you are always behind and never keeping up with those around you? Do you feel out of sync?

7. Do you feel Irritable or have angry feelings frequently?

8. Do you act out with reckless driving or do you take part in dangerous, daredevil activities where you or someone else is at risk?

9. Are you often overwhelmed by simple things or things that are beyond your control?

Are these things that you can identify with? If so, you are most likely under too much stress. It is optimal to rid yourself of as much stress as you possibly can so that your body can begin to take charge over illness and disease. Even if you cannot eliminate all of your stress, do what you can to get rid of what you can.

If you would like to eliminate or at least reduce the stress you have in your life, you will find some helpful hints and tips below. The more you can wipe stress from your life, the more your body can fight against things that can attack it. That does not mean you will never get sick, of course. But you are sure to get sick far less often if you can do some things to reduce your stress level.

- **Exercise daily.** It doesn't require dashing through a marathon to reap the rewards of exercise. Simply doing some activity for 15 minutes a day will help. Exercise is one thing that is terrific for your immune system so be sure and get what you can of it.

- **Plan your day in advance.** Thinking and planning ahead reduces the last minute panic you feel when you have not completed a task. If you are well prepared for what lies ahead, you will be more at ease and you may get to catch a little more sleep as well since you won't have to get up early to finish what you didn't complete the day before.

- **Prioritize and Organize.** When you don't plan properly, you end up with too much on your plate. It is a weight to think of all you have to do and sometimes it is just too much. This stresses you out and stress leads to poor health and poor health gives way to illness and disease. The better you plan and organize, the better off your life will be. You will carry around less stress and you will most likely get more sleep too. Take 30 minutes out of the day to prioritize and organize and you will see a huge difference right off. If you are lacking in organizational skills, recruit the assistance of someone who is good at it like a family member, co-worker or friend. You can also find information on the subject online.

- **Soul Search.** Knowing why you do what you do can lead to solutions. Do you over-stretch yourself because you feel obligated? Do you feel you must take on a mountain load of tasks to feel adequate? Maybe your personality is just one that is inclined to sway to the negative. If so, you may need to work a little harder than most on becoming positive but it can certainly be accomplished.

There are a myriad of ways in which you can cut down on stress.
- Taking a walk is great to reduce stress and anxiety.
- 15 mintute power nap
- Focus on the positive instead of the negative
- Get a massage
- Get a pedicure

- Play with your pet
- Go for a drive in the country
- Drink hot tea
- Take a walk
- Have sex
- Meditate
- Breathe deep
- And more…

The important thing is you find out what works for you. When you notice you become stressed…be aware of it and take charge.

When you stress less, you will not be releasing the dangerous stress hormone and therefore will enable your body to take on more of what it needs to take on like fighting off disease.

Starting a bedtime routine

A bedtime routine is important in getting a good night's rest. You may opt for satin sheets that make you feel relaxed or you may like reading a great book or watching a certain television program. Do what you can to get in the mood for a good night's sleep.

SECRETS OF A GOOD NIGHTS SLEEP

When it comes to helping your body, sleep is one of the very best things you can do for it. If you are not getting the rest you need, you are going to be more likely to catch things like colds, the flu, viruses and bacterial infections. You will also suffer from chronic fatigue. Lack of sleep adds up to a compromised immune system. There are ways that you can improve your sleep though.

Common things that contribute to Sleep Problems

It is common to have issues falling asleep or staying asleep once you do finally crash out. Here are some reasons some have trouble getting to sleep:

1. **Over Obligated**. Some of us have too many things going on which makes it near impossible to get enough rest. Perhaps you have to work two jobs in order to survive financially. The same person telling you that you must get more sleep may be the same person knocking on your door to collect rent. When you are burning the candle at both ends, it takes a toll. Do your best

to narrow down the things you must do and those that may be unnecessary.

2. **Too much on your mind.** When your mind is going nintety-to-nothing, it is difficult to go to sleep. You think of things like what you need to do the next day or what you have done that day. A journal is a good way to productively go over these things, release them and start anew. In order to rest, you need to put all your cares to rest as well.

3. **Watching television in bed.** It's not a good idea to watch television in bed nor is it a good idea to work from bed. The more the bed is associated with sleep, the better. Besides, the energy that comes from the electronic devices such as a television or computer is very likely to make your body unable to relax. When the television is playing, the light actually tells your brain that it is time to rise which can lead to a less than restful sleep if you get any at all.

4. **Drinking prior to bed.** It's a bad idea to drink before bedtime, alcohol especially. It takes about 4 hours to get it out of your system so you can sleep properly. You will notice that you sleep much better when you don't drink awhile before bed and that includes caffeinated beverages as well. .

5. **Exercising right before bedtime.** Exercise is best done first thing in the morning because it boosts your metabolism and stimulates your mind and body. If possible, avoid exercising in the hours just before going to sleep or you may find yourself more awake that you want to be.

Different people require different amounts of sleep. The common amount is 7-8 hours of sleep per night but some people are fine with only 6-7 hours while other need 8-9 hours. Your body will let you know if you tune into it and when it does, it is best to follow its cue. It is necessary to get whatever amount of sleep you body is asking for. That way you can function at your best all day.

Our bodies are able to do miraculous things when we get adequate sleep. We can handle stress and fight disease. You will be much less likely to catch a cold or get an infection when you are caught up on your sleep. Being well rested is powerful so don't underestimate what a good night of it can do. If you are sick or feel like you are fighting getting sick, get even more sleep and you will bounce back much quicker.

If this is the case, you need desperately to catch some sleep. If you have to, call in sick to work. The truth is that you are well on your way to being sick and you will be doing yourself and others a favor. Most work places and bosses would prefer for you to come in at your best after some good rest than to sit on the clock unproductively. Plus, you may be a danger to yourself and to those around you. You certainly stand a chance for catching diseases that you can spread because your immunities are down so low when you are sleep deprived. So, take it to heart and realize that sleep is that important.

You are now more familiar with sleep and are equipped with some tools to help you get more quality sleep. Now let's take a look at some frequently asked questions about elevating your immune system and enabling your body to better fight disease.

Conclusion

Way to go. Congratulations are in order! Now, you are well on your way to living a healthy life and boosting your immune system. Actively taking care of your body is a huge step to wellness and an excellent quality of life. You only get one chance to do it right so take care of your body and it will take care of you.

It is common for people to get sick in winter and spring which can often be attributed to viral infections or allergies. Don't forget to get a bi-annual physical around these times of the year so that you can be sure your body is working at its finest. Remember the helpful pointers and the steps in this guide and you will be on your way to living well and feeling great.

All the best,
Nora Roth

P.S. I sincerely hope you have found immense value in this book. So many people struggle with a weakened immune system and I felt it was very important to share these immune boosting secrets with the word to solve that problem. If you have enjoyed my book please let others know by leaving my book an honest and sincere review on Amazon.

Made in the USA
Lexington, KY
25 April 2016